Caregiver's Guide

To

Prostate Cancer

Gilbert Predmore

"Remember, you're not alone. There are many other caregivers out there who understand what you're going through.
Reach out for support when you need it".

Table of contents

For the
world's caregivers
and the
loved ones
they treasure ...

Introduction

When cancer hits, it has an enormous impact on the patient's life as well as the lives of those who provide care for them. This path may be emotionally and practically overwhelming for the millions of carers who are pushed into the difficult position of assisting a loved one with prostate cancer. We start on a sympathetic investigation of this journey in "A Caregiver's Guide to Prostate Cancer," providing direction, understanding, and empowerment to those who find themselves in this crucial position.

The most prevalent disease in males is prostate cancer, which is diagnosed in millions of new cases each year. It's a condition that may take many different forms and have an impact on a patient's mental health as well as their physical health and the dynamics of their relationships. As carers, you play a crucial role by offering not just physical care but also emotional support, advocacy, and stability in the face of adversity.

The goal of this book is to provide caregivers with the information, resources, and techniques necessary to successfully negotiate the challenges of providing care for men with prostate cancer. We shall explore the disease's medical elements over its pages, demystifying terms and available treatments. But we won't stop there; we'll also examine the emotional landscape of caring to better assist you comprehend the emotional rollercoaster that often comes along with this duty.

We will discuss the victories, tribulations, and priceless lessons learned by actual caregivers and patients. We want to provide you with a complete understanding of the caring for prostate cancer by drawing on professional guidance, recent research, and the collective experience of individuals who have traveled this route.

Our objective is to equip you, the caregiver, with information, empathy, and resilience. We'll provide helpful pointers for dealing with day-to-day difficulties, suggestions for preserving your own wellbeing, and suggestions for promoting open communication with your loved one and the medical staff.

Remember that you are not alone as you begin this road of caring. The book "A Caregiver's Guide to Prostate Cancer" is here to be your friend, your guide, and your pillar of support. This book will be your go-to resource for giving the finest care while protecting your own wellbeing, whether you're a partner, kid, friend, or anyone else taking on the role of caregiver.

Together, we'll go through the ups and downs of providing care for a loved one with prostate cancer, making sure that you, the unsung heroes in this fight, have the information and encouragement you need to be the unwavering pillars of strength that your family members deserve.

I

"Don't be afraid to ask for help. There are many resources available to caregivers, and you don't have to go through this alone."

Prostate Cancer Discussed

Understanding a person's vulnerability to the illness and early identification of prostate cancer depend on knowing the risk factors for the disease. The majority of cases affect males over 50, with age being a key risk factor. Regular screening may assist in identifying prostate cancer at an earlier, more curable stage, particularly in older men. Regular tests may be advised for people who have a family history of prostate cancer since it may raise risk.

Prostate cancer is more frequent in African American males and less common in Asian and Hispanic men, making race/ethnicity another important risk factor. For anyone with a family history of certain mutations, genetic testing and counseling may be advised. A increased risk of prostate cancer is linked to poor food habits, obesity, and inactivity. In addition to improving general health, quitting smoking may lower this risk.

Prostate cancer risk may also be increased by environmental factors including exposure to certain chemicals and pollutants. For people in high-risk professions, occupational exposure should be taken into account. Regular PSA testing and digital rectal examinations (DREs) may help discover prostate cancer in its early stages and improve treatment results. Screening history can also have an impact on early identification.

Making educated choices regarding prostate cancer screening and prevention requires an understanding of these risk factors and their importance for both patients and healthcare professionals. To choose the best strategy for early identification and treatment, men must review their risk factors and screening choices with their healthcare providers.

There are many techniques used for prostate cancer screening, and each has advantages and disadvantages. The PSA Test, Digital Rectal Exam, Multiparametric Magnetic Resonance Imaging (mpMRI), Prostate Biopsy, Risk Assessment Tools, and other biomarkers are the main screening techniques. Each technique has advantages and disadvantages, so it's important for men to talk to their healthcare providers about their risk factors and screening choices in order to choose the best course of action for early identification and therapy.

Individual risk factors, preferences, and talks with a healthcare practitioner all play a role in the technique of prostate cancer screening that is selected. It is critical to weigh the possible advantages and drawbacks of each approach and to include the patient and their healthcare practitioner in the decision-making process. Prostate cancer prevention and early diagnosis depend heavily on routine checkups and PSA (Prostate-Specific Antigen) testing. Prostate cancer is more treatable and perhaps curable when it is discovered early, when it is often asymptomatic, thanks to PSA testing.
Another crucial component of prostate cancer screening is risk assessment. Increased PSA levels may signal the existence of prostate problems and call for more testing. PSA tests aid in risk stratification by directing the frequency and extent of subsequent testing and monitoring. Regular physicals and PSA testing also provide the added

advantage of providing personalized screening. Based on a patient's risk factors, family history, and test findings, healthcare professionals may customize their screening recommendations.

The baseline measurement is crucial for comparison purposes in the future. PSA levels that fluctuate over time may be a better indicator of possible problems. PSA testing is useful in detecting aggressive types of prostate cancer that need immediate action, but it may result in overdiagnosis and overtreatment of indolent tumours. To make decisions that are consistent with their beliefs and interests, people need to be well-informed.

Prostate cancer risk is significantly influenced by genetics. An individual's risk profile is influenced by a number of variables, including family history, inherited gene mutations, other genetic polymorphisms, ethnic and racial characteristics, and polygenic risk scores. Understanding these elements may have practical repercussions for family planning, preventative measures, screening, and treatment choices.

Overall, genetics significantly influences prostate cancer risk, and knowledge of a person's genetic susceptibility may assist inform individualized healthcare choices, such as screening and preventative methods. For those who have a significant family history of prostate cancer or known genetic abnormalities, genetic counseling may be advised in order to determine their particular risk and make wise decisions.

Coping mechanisms are crucial for the treatment and recovery process since a prostate cancer diagnosis may result in serious psychological and emotional difficulties for the patient. These difficulties include social isolation, shock and denial, worry and dread, depression, and body image and sexual problems.

People can seek support from a support network, keep lines of communication open with healthcare professionals, practice mindfulness and relaxation techniques, seek professional assistance, educate themselves about prostate cancer, maintain a healthy lifestyle, support relationships, prioritize self-care activities, set achievable goals, and advocate for their healthcare needs and preferences to cope with these challenges.

Finding the ideal blend of coping tactics may take some time, however, since dealing with prostate cancer is a very unique process. It's completely acceptable to seek expert advice when necessary, and the assistance of family members and medical professionals may be quite helpful all along the way.

Prostate cancer research developments as of September 2021 have resulted in a number of interesting areas of study and their potential influence on future therapies. Researchers have been able to develop more focused medicines and individualized treatment plans by better understanding the genetic abnormalities that cause prostate cancer thanks to advances in genomic profiling and precision medicine. Prostate cancer has showed potential to be treated with immunotherapy, particularly immune checkpoint inhibitors. Research is now being done to improve immunotherapy methods to make them more successful against prostate cancer.

To stop the development of some prostate cancer-related biological targets and signaling pathways, targeted treatments have been created and tried. Stereotactic body radiation treatment (SBRT) and proton therapy are two examples of recent developments in radiotherapy that attempt to provide greater radiation doses to the tumor while avoiding harm to nearby healthy tissue. For more precise diagnosis and focused treatment, PSMA-specific imaging and therapy, including radioligand treatments, are being developed. By analyzing circulating tumor DNA and other biomarkers in blood or urine, liquid biopsy methods provide non-invasive surveillance of the course of the illness and the effectiveness of therapy.

To enhance early detection, diagnosis, and treatment planning for prostate cancer, artificial intelligence (AI) and machine learning are being used to evaluate complex datasets, including medical imaging and genetic data. In order to enhance treatment success, combination treatments investigate the blending of several treatment techniques, including surgery, radiation, chemotherapy, immunotherapy, and targeted therapy. Modern treatments are available because to continuous clinical studies investigating innovative medications and treatment philosophies for prostate cancer.

By minimizing treatment-related side effects, side effect management research seeks to enhance the quality of life for prostate cancer survivors. It's important to keep in mind that not all research findings translate into effective therapies, and that rigorous testing and validation are necessary before new treatments become standard of care. This is because prostate cancer treatment currently lacks effective, targeted, and personalized approaches.

It's advised to check contemporary medical literature, dependable healthcare sources, or chat with a medical oncologist who specializes in prostate cancer for the most recent information about developments in prostate cancer research and their effects on therapies.

Prostate cancer risk may be strongly influenced by lifestyle choices including food and exercise. By supplying vital vitamins, minerals, and antioxidants, a plant-based diet high in fruits, vegetables, whole grains, tomatoes, and lycopene may reduce the risk of prostate cancer. Prostate cancer risk may also be decreased by eating less processed food and sweets as well as fatty fish and soy products.

Regular exercise may help you maintain a healthy weight and lower your chances of developing prostate cancer. It's important to maintain a healthy weight since obesity raises the chance of developing aggressive prostate cancer. Exercises that increase muscle mass and general fitness may help with weight control. For better health overall, it's also crucial to cut down on inactive time.

Moderate alcohol intake, quitting smoking, and routine prostate cancer screening are other lifestyle choices that may help lower the risk of prostate cancer. Prostate cancer risk is also influenced by genetics and other variables. Prostate cancer risk may be decreased with a balanced strategy that includes a nutritious diet, frequent exercise, and other healthy lifestyle choices.

The use of the PSA (Prostate-Specific Antigen) test as a prostate cancer screening tool has generated discussion and disagreement in the medical profession. Since the test may identify prostate cancer at an early stage yet not all prostate tumors are severe or life-threatening, there is some debate over the potential for overdiagnosis and overtreatment. Critics claim that this results in overtreating tumors that are sluggish.

Lacking specificity, the PSA test is unable to accurately discriminate between tumors that are aggressive and those that are not. This may cause patients' worry and unneeded biopsies. The test also lacks specificity, making it impossible to accurately discriminate between tumors that are aggressive and those that are not. Prostate biopsies, which are often carried out in response to a high PSA test, may be harmful and vary across recommendations, which may result in consequences including bleeding and infection.

Numerous PSA tests may not have significantly decreased prostate cancer mortality, according to some research. The advantage in terms of lowering fatalities due to prostate cancer is still up for debate. Concerns about the cost-effectiveness of PSA testing have been raised since it may increase healthcare expenses without clearly improving outcomes or survival rates.

The importance of shared decision-making between patients and healthcare professionals is rising. This involves talking about the possible advantages and disadvantages of PSA screening and empowering individuals to make educated decisions based on their unique risk factors and beliefs. Considering a man's age, risk factors, and preferences when deciding whether to undergo PSA testing and how regularly to do so has become increasingly commonplace in recent years as a result of these concerns. Other instruments are being utilized to direct choices for prostate cancer screening and follow-up, such as risk calculators and cutting-edge imaging methods like mpMRI.

Treatment and Side Effect

Options for treating prostate cancer differ depending on the condition's stage, aggressiveness, general health of the patient, and personal preferences. Active monitoring, surgery, radiation therapy, hormone therapy, chemotherapy, immunotherapy, targeted therapy, cryotherapy, and high-intensity focused ultrasound (HIFU) are common forms of treatment.

In order to help a loved one throughout the decision-making process, caregivers are essential. They help with medical visits, provide information, and offer emotional support. They support decision-making, coordinate treatment, and speak out for their loved one's preferences within the healthcare system. In order to choose the optimal course of therapy, they suggest getting a second opinion. During therapy, they help with practical requirements and everyday duties including food preparation and transportation.

Because choices about prostate cancer therapy may be very personal, it is crucial to respect autonomy. The caregiver's job is to help and enlighten the patient while honoring their autonomy and preferences.

There are many different prostate cancer treatment choices available depending on the stage, aggressiveness, general health of the patient, and personal preferences. In order to assist and enlighten patients while upholding their autonomy and choices, caregivers play a crucial role.

Treatments for prostate cancer may have a variety of adverse effects, whose severity varies from person to person. Incontinence, radiation, hormone treatment, chemotherapy, immunotherapy and targeted therapy, cryotherapy and HIFU, as well as swelling, pain, and urine symptoms are examples of common side effects. Incontinence products, pelvic floor exercises, and emotional support for intimacy problems should all be provided by caregivers.

The side effects of radiation treatment include gastrointestinal abnormalities, urinary issues, and exhaustion. Hot flashes, a drop in libido, mood changes, muscle loss, and exhaustion may all be side effects of hormone treatment. Creating a comfortable atmosphere for hot flashes, giving emotional support for mood swings, promoting a balanced diet and regular exercise, and addressing interpersonal issues are all good caregiver ideas.

Chemotherapy may result in tiredness, hair loss, nausea, vomiting, and an elevated risk of infections. To lower the risk of infection, caregivers should assist with food preparation, hydration, wig choosing or head coverings, and maintaining a clean and hygienic environment. Fatigue, skin responses, gastrointestinal problems, and immune-related side effects are all potential consequences of immunotherapy and targeted treatment. In addition to helping with skincare, caregivers should alter food to treat gastrointestinal issues and watch out for any immune-related adverse effects.

Swelling, pain, and urinary symptoms may be brought on by HIFU and cryotherapy. The management of urinary symptoms and comfort measures should all be provided by caregivers.

Keeping lines of communication open with the medical staff, fostering mental well-being, controlling medication, encouraging a balanced diet and exercise regimen, and looking for help from support groups are all general advice for carers.

To better support their loved one's choices and interact with medical experts, caregivers should be aware about prostate cancer, treatment options, and possible side effects. Open lines of communication are essential, and accompanying the patient to medical visits may assist to make sure all concerns are addressed and provide emotional support.

Stress and uncertainty may be reduced by fostering a supportive atmosphere at home, encouraging emotional support, advocating for self-care, being adaptable, encouraging healthy habits, having a positive perspective, respecting autonomy, looking for support groups, and assisting patients with future planning.
In summary,every caregiver's experience is different, and what works best for them relies on their capacity to provide their loved one with prostate cancer treatment with emotional support, practical help, and flexibility.

Both patients and caregivers may have severe emotional and psychological effects as a result of prostate cancer. Due to the course of the illness and the effectiveness of therapy, patients may suffer dread, worry, sadness, loss of identity, and uncertainty. Aside from emotional tiredness, caregivers may also suffer worry, anxiety, guilt, and other negative emotions as a result of having to accompany a loved one during cancer treatment.

In order to offer emotional support to patients during treatment, caregivers should actively listen to their worries, encourage expression, encourage self-care, be patient, stay informed about the disease and available treatments, celebrate small victories, offer reassurance, share responsibilities, and organize relaxing activities. While enabling patients to share their emotions and have their feelings validated, active listening may be calming and comforting.

Additionally, caregivers need to be patient and sympathetic while dealing with mood swings or emotional ups and downs. It may be important to seek professional assistance if the patient or caregiver experiences extreme emotional discomfort. Maintaining a good mindset and boosting morale may be accomplished through delivering comfort and celebrating little accomplishments. Both patients and caregivers might benefit emotionally by scheduling downtime and sharing chores in order to avoid fatigue.

Prostate cancer treatment may be emotionally taxing, but patients and caregivers can travel this path together with the correct emotional support. The mental health of both partners may be greatly enhanced by developing a solid support system and getting expert help.

Diet and nutrition are essential for controlling the negative effects of prostate cancer therapy. A healthy diet may improve overall health and aid in the relief of certain treatment-related symptoms. A combination of carbs, proteins, and healthy fats may help control side effects including nausea and vomiting from chemotherapy, diarrhea from radiation treatment or certain drugs, constipation from pain medications or inactivity, and lack of appetite.
Caretakers should make sure the patient drinks enough of fluids, consumes foods high in antioxidants, concentrates on lean proteins, incorporates healthy fats, maintains calcium and vitamin D levels, and advocates a diet high in fiber to support general health. Lycopene-rich foods, limiting red meat consumption, consuming soy in moderation, and staying hydrated are some special dietary concerns.

During prostate cancer therapy, effective communication is crucial between caregivers, patients, and medical professionals for a number of reasons. Making choices regarding treatment is made possible by effective communication, which guarantees that patients and caregivers completely comprehend the diagnosis, available treatments, potential risks, and benefits. When patients fully understand their treatment regimens and have access to their healthcare professionals to address any concerns or side effects, they are more likely to follow them. By allowing patients and caregivers to communicate their worries, anxieties, and emotional needs, emotional support helps create a helpful atmosphere during a trying time.

Attending doctor's meetings, preparing questions, serving as a liaison, advocating for the patient, maintaining records, promoting candor, requesting clarity, using technology, respecting privacy, and getting second views are all ways that caregivers may promote good communication.

In summary, treating the adverse effects of prostate cancer therapy requires a well-balanced diet, efficient communication, and an awareness of individual dietary demands. Caretakers may assist patients in overcoming the difficulties of prostate cancer therapy and preserving their general wellbeing by adhering to these recommendations.

During their journey of providing care, caregivers of men with prostate cancer may encounter a variety of difficulties and anxieties. These include the emotional toll, coping with the course of therapy, risk, self-sacrifice, physical demands, and financial pressure. In order to overcome these difficulties, carers must put their own health first, enlist the help of friends and family, practice relaxing methods, and take pauses to refuel.

Caregivers may join support groups to connect with others facing similar issues and share experiences, obstacles, and coping mechanisms. Essential coping mechanisms for carers include delegation of responsibilities, open communication, realistic expectations, professional assistance when required, financial preparation, respite care, preparing for the future, organization, and acknowledging minor victories.

For carers of men with prostate cancer, self-care is essential because it promotes mental and physical well-being, improves caring, and enables them to continue in that position for an extended period of time. Setting boundaries, asking for help when necessary, seeking professional support, planning short breaks, scheduling regular health checkups, incorporating exercise into routines, establishing a regular sleep schedule, practicing relaxation techniques, engaging in hobbies and interests, time management, learning about prostate cancer and its treatment, and staying informed on available curative means.

The following tips will better guide you as a caregiver;

1. **Establish boundaries:** Clearly identify your job as a caregiver and let other family members, friends, and medical professionals know where you draw the line. Recognize when to say no.

2. **Seek help:Share** your thoughts and emotions with friends, family, or support groups.

3. To keep track of your physical and emotional health, make regular appointments with your healthcare professional.

4. Include physical activity in your daily routine, even if it's only little strolls or easy workouts, to reduce stress and increase vitality.

5. Keep up a healthy eating regimen and stay away from sweets and caffeine in excess since these might cause energy dumps.

6. Make sleep a priority and create a regular sleep regimen.

7. Use relaxation methods to lower stress and enhance emotional well-being, such as deep breathing, mindfulness, or meditation.

8. **Take part in interests and hobbies:** Schedule time for leisure pursuits that will provide you a much-needed break from caring duties.

9. **Time management:** Plan your caregiving tasks so that you have time for your own obligations and leisure time.

10. **approach for assistance:** If you ever need it, don't be afraid to approach your friends or other family members for support. In order to lessen the burden, assign tasks.

12. Take into account going to counseling or therapy to deal with any emotional difficulties or stress related to caring.

13. Become knowledgeable about prostate cancer and its treatment to better comprehend the requirements of patients and their medical journeys.

14. **Keep yourself informed:** Stay current on local and online caregiver information and support services.

In conclusion, carers of men with prostate cancer must overcome a variety of obstacles and use coping mechanisms to maintain their own well-being and the kind of care they provide. Caregivers may provide their loved ones the greatest support and care possible by prioritizing their own well-being, getting expert assistance, and being educated.

The wellbeing of carers and the people they care for depends on self-care. Support groups and services that are suited to their requirements may be helpful to caregivers by offering them emotional support, knowledge, and a feeling of community. Caregiver-specific organizations, cancer centers, online resources, social media platforms, local support groups, community centers, medical social workers, medical professionals, healthcare facilities, national cancer support lines, online support apps, and professional counseling services can all offer caregivers helpful information and support.

The long-term effects of prostate cancer therapy on patients and carers should be understood by caregivers. Physical side effects that patients may suffer include weariness, incontinence, and erectile dysfunction might affect their quality of life and self-esteem. Prostate cancer patients may continue to experience anxiety, despair, or worry of cancer recurrence even after their treatment is over. In the post-treatment period, routine follow-up checkups and continuing monitoring are typical to look for any indications of cancer recurrence or long-term adverse effects. Additionally, there may be other adverse effects and long-term health implications associated with hormone treatment.

After providing care, caregivers may endure emotional hangover, adjustment, relational alterations, ongoing self-care needs, and identity struggles. They may need some time to get used to their new situation, reestablish and redefine connections, and put their own well-being first. After finishing their caring duties, caregivers may have identity issues, particularly if caregiving occupied a significant portion of their lives for a long time.

In order to get ready for the post-treatment phase, caregivers can stay in constant contact with the patient about their physical and emotional well-being, foster a supportive environment, ensure that they attend scheduled follow-up appointments, continue self-care practices, reevaluate their goals and priorities, stay in touch with support networks, and be ready for any potential ups and downs as they adjust to life after treatment. The trick is to be patient and flexible.

Active therapy for prostate cancer does not always spell the end of it. As the patient and family navigate the post-treatment period, caregivers should be ready for the long-term effects and continue to provide support, both emotionally and practically. Caregivers who prioritize their own needs may better address the needs of their loved ones while preserving their own well-being and resiliency throughout the caring process.

Beginning of A Caregiver's Journey

When a loved one receives a prostate cancer diagnosis, a range of complicated feelings and ideas may arise. There could be initial shock and disbelief, then dread and worry about the future. People often experience intense stress about the treatment procedure and its consequences, as well as a great feeling of care for the wellbeing of their loved one. A person may wonder why this occurred or look for information about prostate cancer and its therapies. Additionally, there can be a desire to provide the individual receiving the diagnosis emotional support and useful aid.

Common emotions include grief, rage, and helplessness, but they may also include optimism and a desire to unite in the battle against the illness. To go through this difficult journey, it's critical for the person with the diagnosis and their loved ones to reach out for support, be honest with one another, and work together.

Consider taking the following actions to learn more and comprehend your available treatment options:

1. **Speak with medical experts:** Arrange a meeting with the physician who made the diagnosis

and inquire about the cancer's stage, prognosis, and suggested therapies.

2. **Get a second opinion:** Take into account seeking a second opinion from a different doctor or expert. You may make an educated choice by considering the many viewpoints and treatment suggestions that various physicians may have.

3. **Online research:** To learn more about prostate cancer, its phases, and available treatments, consult reliable sources like the websites of cancer organizations (such as the American Cancer Society and Cancer Research UK). Be wary of false information.

4. **Join a nearby or online support group for men with prostate cancer:** Join a nearby or online support group for men with prostate cancer.

5. **Speak with survivors:** Make contact with others who have overcome prostate cancer or who have had comparable medical procedures. Their knowledge and experiences may be quite helpful in figuring out what to anticipate throughout treatment and recovery.

6. Examine the treatments and services covered by your loved one's health insurance coverage to learn more.

7. Look for institutions or clinics that specialize in the treatment of prostate cancer. Think about obtaining care in a facility with a dedicated cancer center.

8. **Keep records of all information:** Keep tabs on doctor's notes, test results, and treatment schedules.

9. **Seek emotional support:** Don't forget to look out for your own and your loved one's mental health. To deal with the emotional difficulties that often accompany a cancer diagnosis, seek counseling or therapy.

10. **Involve the patient:** Do your best to involve your loved one in these conversations.

It may be emotionally difficult to discuss a loved one's prostate cancer diagnosis and treatment options with them. These difficulties may be overcome by balancing candor with compassion, comprehending medical language, negotiating treatment choices, supporting autonomy, coping with ambiguity, managing family dynamics, talking about the practical elements of therapy, and overcoming feelings of burden.

The first step in helping your loved one with prostate cancer is to find the best doctors, nurses, and experts. Start by speaking with your primary care physician, who may recommend experts depending on the diagnosis and your particular need. It is often beneficial to get second views since they might provide more information and treatment choices. Consider seeking treatment in a cancer center or hospital with a specialized cancer department, and do your homework on the qualifications and expertise of possible healthcare providers, such as urologists or oncologists who are board certified.

To confirm that the chosen healthcare providers are in-network, which may greatly impact the cost of treatment, check your loved one's health insurance coverage. Set up consultations with possible experts to go through treatment choices, evaluate the doctor's communication skills, and determine if the doctor is prepared to engage you and your loved one in the decision-making process. Inquire about referrals from cancer-care-experienced friends, family members, or support groups.

Depending on the stage and kind of prostate cancer, you may want to consider radiation oncology or surgery oncology as treatment options. Make sure the medical staff you choose has the capacity to handle all parts of the required care. Make sure your loved one feels comfortable speaking honestly about their concerns, treatment preferences, and anxieties by assessing the relationship between them and the medical staff.

Continuous assessment is necessary to guarantee that you can reevaluate and switch healthcare providers if you're unhappy with the care or if circumstances change while you're receiving treatment. Making educated judgments and delivering the best possible care and support depend on having open lines of communication with the experts of choice, getting second views, and being knowledgeable about the available treatments.

Taking on caregiving responsibilities once a loved one is diagnosed with prostate cancer is crucial to supporting their journey. Initial tasks that frequently need to be completed include making plans for appointments, gathering medical information, looking into treatment options, making a medication schedule, managing appointments, taking notes, offering emotional support, keeping track of dietary requirements, exercising and engaging in physical activity, managing insurance and finances, finding friends and family who can offer help and emotional support, and setting aside time for self-care.

The road that might include continuing care and assistance is just getting started with these basic caregiving duties. Being prepared, knowledgeable, and attentive to your loved one's needs is vital. You should also seek out assistance from support networks and healthcare experts as necessary.

When taking care of someone with prostate cancer, creating a support system is essential. This network consists of close relatives, close friends, support groups, medical professionals, therapists, and counselors as well as employers, respite care providers, volunteer groups, financial and legal advisers, spiritual or religious communities, internet resources, and home healthcare providers.

The network of support gave them emotional sturdiness, shared accountability, and useful aid. It was a team effort involving several people and resources. Over time, the author came to understand that asking for assistance and relying on this network was not a sign of weakness but rather an essential step in rendering the finest care while preserving one's own wellbeing.

Prostate cancer caregiving often necessitates considerable daily routine modifications. A flexible work schedule, prioritizing time management, setting boundaries, daily planning, a self-care routine, healthy eating, a support network, communication, delegation, financial planning, an adaptable mindset, educational efforts, and staying informed about the condition and treatment plan are some lifestyle modifications and adjustments that the author made to accommodate caregiving responsibilities.

Early on in a patient's care for prostate cancer, emotional support and self-care are essential. By acting as a safety net, emotional support soothes, lessens loneliness, encourages honest conversation, validates emotions, and lessens stress. In order to avoid burnout, maintain physical health, seek treatment or counseling when necessary, manage time effectively, create boundaries, get support, build coping mechanisms, and preserve identity, self-care is crucial.

Careful preparation, flexibility, and support are necessary to successfully juggle caregiving responsibilities with personal and professional life. Prioritize and schedule caring duties based on urgency and significance, provide time for personal and professional responsibilities, and be transparent with your employer about your caregiving position and any possible need for schedule flexibility. It is easier to manage the workload when tasks like grocery shopping, food preparation, and transportation to appointments are shared and delegated.

Regular exercise, a nutritious diet, and enough sleep are all important components of self-care for preserving one's physical and mental wellbeing. It's also crucial to schedule leisure time, hobbies, and things that make you happy and relieve tension. By discussing their caring obligations with their managers and HR departments, investigating flexible work schedules and extra help if required, and seeking advice from Employee Assistance Programs (EAPs) or counseling services offered by their workplace, caregivers may get professional support.

Options for respite care provide momentary relaxation from caring duties, enabling carers to concentrate on personal and professional obligations without feeling overburdened. They discuss their caregiving strategy jointly and must be open with loved ones about their wants and limits.

Caregiving obligations may be unexpected, so carers must be flexible and adaptable. Caregivers should maintain their flexibility and make necessary scheduling adjustments. Setting limits is crucial because it enables them to decline extra obligations that can compromise their capacity to provide high-quality care.

Last but not least, a support system, which includes friends and family, offers emotional support and aid with caregiving duties, acting as a safety net when necessary. Caregivers might better prepare for the difficulties that lie ahead in the caring journey by paying priority to these elements.

The author discusses their experience juggling caring, a personal life, and a career while undergoing early prostate cancer therapy. They stress the need of taking care of oneself, asking for help when necessary, and keeping lines of communication open with family members and coworkers.

The author offers the following significant suggestions for caregivers:

1. To make wise choices and assist your loved one successfully, educate yourself about prostate cancer, its stages, treatment options, and possible side effects.

2. To learn about various viewpoints and treatment alternatives, get second opinions from several healthcare providers.

3. Promote open dialogue with your loved one and let them voice their worries, preferences, and anxieties.

4. Create a support system by contacting caregiver support groups for prostate cancer patients.

5. Take care of yourself since caregivers often overlook their own health. Give yourself a high priority.

6. Recognize that asking for assistance from friends and family is an essential step in the caring process.

7. Speak up for your loved one's medical needs by enquiring and getting more information.

8. Recognize the cost of prostate cancer treatment, examine insurance coverage, look into financial help options, and make a budget to handle medical costs.

9. Obtain expert counseling or treatment to be ready for emotional difficulties.

10. Proceed cautiously and divide the trip into small chunks.

11. Commemorate little successes and landmarks in your loved one's medical journey to provide encouragement and hope at trying moments.

12. Maintain meticulous records of your health-related information, prescriptions, and appointments for future consultation with medical specialists.

13. Make future plans and, if necessary, talk to your loved one about advance directives and end-of-life care.

14. Strike a good balance between your connections with family and friends and your caring obligations.

15. Be optimistic; prostate cancer therapies are improving, and your commitment is priceless.

"Being a caregiver is a tough job, but it's also one of the most rewarding. You're making a difference in someone's life, and that's something to be proud of"

Specific Tasks and Challenges

Due to a number of variables, caring for a loved one who has prostate cancer may be emotionally taxing. The following are some of them: fear and worry, doubt about the cancer diagnosis and its course, role adjustment, guilt and self-criticism, loss of independence, loneliness, depression and burnout, communication difficulties, loss and bereavement, and resentment. Caregivers can emphasize self-care, establish boundaries, seek assistance from friends, family, support groups, and healthcare experts to help them deal with these emotional difficulties. They should also be transparent with their loved one and the healthcare team.

For a number of reasons, communication between caregivers and medical experts is essential. Effective communication makes ensuring that caregivers are aware of the prostate cancer diagnosis, available treatments, and possible side effects, enabling them to offer educated support and collaborate with the medical team on well-informed choices. Caretakers may ensure that prescriptions are taken as directed, appointments are maintained, and treatment plans are followed by keeping open lines of communication. Additionally, caregivers must keep track of any changes in the patient's status and report them so that early action may be made as needed.

Treatment side effects must be carefully handled if prostate cancer may be treated, and caregivers must inform medical professionals of any adverse effects. Changing drugs or therapies may be necessary for this. Medical specialists may provide guidance on how to manage stress, anxiety, and other emotions connected to the patient's illness, so carers also need emotional support.

Multiple healthcare professionals, such as urologists, oncologists, radiologists, and others, who are engaged in a patient's treatment need coordinated care. All healthcare professionals must be informed on the patient's treatment plan and progress in order for effective communication to take place. Caretakers need advocacy because they often act as advocates for the people they love. It is essential for carers to obtain information on the patient's health, available treatments, and available support services. Advanced or terminal cases need end-of-life planning, and conversations regarding palliative care and end-of-life care should include the carers.

Since prostate cancer therapy often entails a continuum of therapies and follow-up care, continuity of care is crucial. The transmission of the patient's medical history and treatment plan between healthcare professionals is made possible through effective communication.

In conclusion, efficient communication between carers and medical professionals is essential to ensure that patients get the best treatment possible, caregivers can carry out their responsibilities successfully, and patients and caregivers receive the emotional support they need throughout the cancer journey. The overall quality of treatment is improved through teamwork and open, honest communication.

The considerable financial obligations and resources accessible to caretakers of men with prostate cancer emphasize the financial cost of caring. Direct medical expenditures, travel expenses, missed wages, out-of-pocket expenses, and the effect on retirement plans may be borne by caregivers. Working with insurance companies to optimize benefits, using government programs like Medicaid, Medicare, and Veterans Affairs, and taking into account nonprofit groups that provide financial help, grants, and support for carers are all ways that caregivers may lessen these financial responsibilities.

In order to help carers combine their employment and caring commitments, employers may also provide caregiver support programs, flexible work schedules, or paid leave choices. Programs for respite care relieve some of the financial and emotional strains on carers by allowing them to take brief breaks while the patient is cared for by qualified specialists. Financial planning services may assist carers in making wise choices about budgeting, investing, and retirement planning both while and after providing care. Support groups may provide both emotional support as well as information on available financial resources and cost-management techniques for caring.

In order to handle the negative effects of therapy for prostate cancer, caregivers are essential. They can monitor symptoms, offer emotional support, manage dietary requirements, help with mobility, provide transportation, keep open lines of communication with the medical staff, encourage activity and exercise, manage pain and incontinence, offer emotional respite, advocate for their loved one's needs within the healthcare system, educate themselves about potential side effects, and more.

To avoid caregiver burnout, caregivers should prioritize their own well-being and get help when necessary. They have to speak out for their loved one's demands inside the medical system, making sure that treatment programs are customized to the patient's particular side effects and worries. They may arm themselves with knowledge about the probable side effects of the particular prostate cancer therapy that their loved one is receiving, allowing them to better predict and manage adverse effects.

Making adjustments to the house to meet physical constraints or offering a peaceful and stress-reducing environment are two examples of creating a pleasant and supportive home environment. Overall, caregivers play a crucial part in improving the quality of life of prostate cancer patients, improving treatment results, and promoting the emotional wellbeing of patients as they manage the difficulties presented by treatment side effects. The secret to successfully managing these side effects is open communication with medical providers and a teamwork-based approach to caring.

Although navigating the healthcare system and fighting for a loved one with prostate cancer may be challenging, doing so is crucial to get the best treatment. Build a care team, communicate clearly, comprehend the treatment plan, ask questions, fight for informed consent, keep thorough records, coordinate care, seek emotional support, deal with financial concerns, be an effective advocate, think about end-of-life care, and take care of yourself if you want to successfully navigate this journey.

Making educated choices and navigating the healthcare system need education. The accuracy of the information may be increased by assembling a team of medical experts with expertise in prostate cancer. Other crucial actions include advocating for informed consent, highlighting risks and benefits, and posing inquiries regarding the treatment plan. To ensure a consistent treatment strategy, thorough records of doctor visits, test findings, prescriptions, and treatment plans must be kept.

Another critical component of caring is managing drugs, which requires watching over schedules, dosages, and any interactions. It might be helpful to coordinate treatment amongst several healthcare practitioners and to get second views from other trained doctors. You may look for emotional assistance via counseling, therapy, or support groups. Consult a financial adviser or social worker to investigate insurance coverage, financial assistance programs, and other financial help sources while dealing with financial issues.

Being an effective advocate means standing up for your loved one's needs and encouraging them to express their worries while being firm yet courteous. When speaking with healthcare professionals, be sure to use clear, precise language. For their intentions to be recorded and honored, it is crucial to discuss end-of-life care and advance directives with your loved one and the medical staff.

Self-care is also crucial for preserving one's physical and mental health. As the course of the therapy develops, your position as an advocate may change. You can contribute to making sure that your loved one has the best treatment possible throughout their prostate cancer journey by remaining informed, speaking clearly, and being proactive.

Role shifts, emotional stress, difficulty communicating, and financial pressure may all be brought on by caregiving, which can have a significant negative influence on family dynamics and relationships. To provide your loved one the greatest care possible, it is crucial to be aware of these obstacles and collaborate.

Caregiving for a man with prostate cancer may have a big influence on family dynamics and relationships, but it can also make families closer and foster traits like empathy, resiliency, and respect for one another. Observation and follow-up care, emotional recovery, treatment side effects, coping with survivorship, enhancing the patient's quality of life, communication with healthcare providers, end-of-life planning, long-term financial planning, relationship adjustments, self-care, support networks, and legacy and reflection can all pose significant long-term challenges and adjustments for caregivers.

In addition to providing emotional support, managing treatment side effects, coping with survivorship, managing changes in physical health, addressing remaining treatment-related concerns, and returning to a more "normal" life, caregivers may also need to monitor and follow up on care. They may also need to concentrate on enhancing the patient's general quality of life, changing the patient's lifestyle, treating any remaining pain or discomfort, and managing chronic symptoms.

In order to advocate for the patient's needs and provide information about the patient's health with healthcare professionals, caregivers may also need to interact with them. For caregivers to successfully traverse these issues, end-of-life preparation, long-term financial planning, relationship modifications, self-care, support networks, and legacy and reflection are crucial.

Caregiver talks concerning hospice, palliative care, and end-of-life care may be necessary in circumstances when prostate cancer is advanced or fatal. Considering continuous medical costs, insurance coverage, and anticipated changes in the patient's capacity to work are all possible components of long-term financial planning.

To avoid burnout, caregivers should put self-care first and strike a balance between their caring duties and personal well-being. Support groups may assist in addressing the emotional and psychological effects of caring, and contemplation on the experience and its effects on one's relationships and other aspects of one's life can help one's loved one's legacy be preserved.

Long-term caring during prostate cancer treatment may be difficult, but caregivers can assist their loved ones' journey into survivorship while preserving their own wellbeing through consistent communication, support, and adaptability.

Dietary modifications and nutritional considerations are essential for the general health and wellbeing of prostate cancer patients. For optimal health, eat a well-balanced diet that is high in fruits, vegetables, whole grains, lean protein, and healthy fats. It strengthens the immune system, supports general health, and helps control adverse effects of medication. Maintaining a balanced diet, making sure the patient keeps hydrated, eating foods rich in fiber, boosting protein consumption, and including omega-3 fatty acids are important factors to take into account.

For good bone health, you should limit your intake of red meat and processed meals, consume foods high in antioxidants, and stay away from foods high in sugar and saturated fats. For healthy bones, particularly if undergoing therapy that alters bone density, it's critical to consume enough calcium and vitamin D. Overindulging in sweets and saturated fats might make it easier to control side effects including nausea, appetite loss, and digestive problems.

It's critical to maintain hydration to prevent aggravating side effects like weariness. Small, frequent meals may aid in the management of digestive problems, appetite loss, and nausea. Before beginning any supplements, get advice from a medical professional or dietician. Depending on the patient's health and treatment requirements, specialized diets—like the Mediterranean diet or a plant-based diet—might be advised.

Meal planning, grocery shopping, portion management, keeping an eye on side effects, encouraging hydration, supporting dietary restrictions, being knowledgeable about nutritional advice, and fostering contact with healthcare professionals are all important caregiver responsibilities. It is crucial to consider the patient's preferences while making meal plans and dietary recommendations. A healthy diet that is well-balanced may help patients recover from prostate cancer therapy and maintain their overall wellbeing.

Prostate cancer therapy must include advance care planning because it enables patients to voice their choices for interventions and treatments while still conveying their desires. This makes it possible to provide individualized care, preserve control, ease the strain on families, prevent conflicts, give priority to quality of life, and provide peace of mind.

By defining their responsibilities in end-of-life decision-making, lessening their emotional load, aligning with the patient's values, enhancing communication, offering support in times of crisis, and placing a priority on quality of life, caregivers may gain from advance care planning. Caregivers who adhere to recorded advance care instructions are also protected legally.

Prostate cancer patients and their caregivers must start the conversation about advance care planning early in the course of the illness, enabling individuals to modify their choices as necessary. Advance care directives may be made more complete and legitimate legally by consulting with legal experts and medical practitioners.

As a caregiver, it may be difficult and confusing to manage several facets of care for people with prostate cancer. several treatment options, a multidisciplinary approach, and several logistical issues are often part of prostate cancer therapy. Medical coordination, treatment decision-making, side effects, medication management, nutrition and diet, logistical coordination, emotional support, advocacy, juggling multiple responsibilities, end-of-life planning, legal and financial considerations, self-care, and coordination with other caregivers are just a few of the challenges that caregivers may encounter.

Medical coordination include communication, scheduling, and appointment-making between various healthcare professionals. Researching and comprehending many treatment choices is necessary for making treatment decisions, and dealing with side effects including exhaustion, incontinence, and sexual dysfunction may be difficult. In order to help the patient deal with these consequences, caregivers must also organize any further medical treatment that may be required.

Medication management include making sure the patient takes their prescriptions as directed and informs healthcare professionals of any negative side effects. Planning and preparation for nutrition and food are crucial for controlling treatment side effects and general health.

Transportation to and from medical visits, handling insurance paperwork, and overseeing financial elements of treatment are all part of logistical coordination. Caretakers have a crucial role in providing comfort and confidence to the patient by providing ongoing emotional support, which is their obligation. Getting second views, making sure the patient's perspective is heard while making treatment choices, and fighting for prompt treatment are all aspects of advocacy.

Stress and burnout may result from juggling commitments like job and family. Self-care, legal and financial considerations, and end-of-life preparation are all difficult but essential components of prostate cancer therapy.

To sum up, prior care planning is crucial for both patients and caregivers to manage the many facets of care associated with treating prostate cancer. Caregivers may overcome these difficulties and provide their loved ones compassionate and dignified care by encouraging efficient communication, a support network, and access to resources.

Resources For Caregivers

The American Cancer Society (ACS) provides a range of organizations and services to assist those who are caring for a loved one who has been diagnosed with prostate cancer. These organizations include the National Cancer Institute (NCI), the Family Caregiver Alliance, the Use TOO International Prostate Cancer Education and Support Network, the Prostate Cancer Foundation (PCF), CancerCare, and the American Cancer Society (ACS).

Another option for carers is to participate in support groups and forums. Websites like Inspire feature vibrant communities where caregivers may interact and exchange experiences. A number of books and articles, like "The Prostate Cancer Dilemma" by Roger S. Kirby and "The Complete Guide to Prostate Cancer: Everything You Need to Know About Diagnosis, Treatment, and Living with Prostate Cancer" by Arnon Krongrad, may provide readers in-depth knowledge on prostate cancer.

Local hospitals and cancer clinics often provide educational courses, counseling services, and caregiver support programs. It is crucial to inquire about resources with nearby medical facilities. Social workers or therapists who focus on cancer care may provide caregivers helpful emotional support and coping mechanisms.

Inspire Prostate Cancer Support Community, PCF Caregiver Group, Cancer Support Community (CSC), HealthUnlocked Prostate Cancer Support Community, Smart Patients Prostate Cancer Community, Reddit Prostate Cancer Community, Facebook Support Groups, and Local Cancer Centers and Hospitals are a few examples of online support groups and communities for caregivers of patients with prostate cancer. When joining, it is important to put online privacy and security first since these communities provide a more private and intimate setting for conversation.

Reaching out to these resources may help caregivers better comprehend and negotiate the road of caring for a loved one with prostate cancer, keeping in mind that caregiving can be both emotionally and physically taxing.

Caregiving for a person with prostate cancer requires managing their food requirements and offering nutritional assistance. Lean proteins, whole grains, fruits, and vegetables are all important components of a balanced diet that may help maintain general health and control the negative effects of medication. Foods high in antioxidants, such berries, tomatoes, and leafy greens, may aid in immune system support and cell protection. Prostate cancer development may be made more likely by limiting red and processed meats. Include omega-3 fatty acids, which are found in fatty fish like salmon, as well as other healthy fats in your diet, such as avocados, almonds, and olive oil. Whole grains, beans, and other fiber-rich meals may improve digestion and lower the risk of constipation.

Make sure your loved one drinks enough water to be hydrated, particularly if they have side symptoms like diarrhea or bladder problems. Limit sugar and processed meals, pay attention to portion management, and be aware of their sensitivity to hot and acidic foods in order to maintain a healthy weight. Before providing them vitamins or herbal treatments, check with their doctor since some of them can conflict with their therapy or medicine.

Create a customized nutrition plan that is tailored to their requirements by speaking with a registered dietitian with expertise in oncology or prostate cancer. Help with meal planning and preparation, and prepare meals in advance to freeze for days when your loved one may not feel like cooking.

Support emotional eating by acknowledging that changes in hunger and eating patterns may result from stress or side effects of medication.

As a caretaker, it may be difficult to manage the adverse effects of prostate cancer treatments, but there are a number of techniques that can be used.

1. Keep yourself up to date on any possible adverse effects of the particular therapy the patient is receiving. Effective caring depends on the patient and their healthcare team having open communication.

2. Follow the patient's doctor-recommended medication regimen and keep note of any dose adjustments.

3. Encourage a healthy diet to help the patient in general. If you want advice on dietary decisions that might help you control side effects, speak with a trained dietitian.

4. Make sure the patient is well hydrated by having water on hand.

5. If the patient's health permits, encourage mild exercise since it may boost mood, vitality, and general well-being.

6. Provide emotional support and patience, keeping in mind that the patient may feel upset owing to side effects.

7. Work with the medical team to manage certain side effects, such as using drugs and other treatments to deal with exhaustion, discomfort, or nausea.

8. Control tiredness by planning rest intervals, setting priorities, and getting help with everyday duties.

9. Join a caregiver support group to connect with people going through similar circumstances and learn coping mechanisms from them.

10. To avoid caregiver fatigue, seek respite care as necessary. Investigate complementary treatments like acupuncture, yoga, or meditation to lessen side effects and anxiety.

11. Adjust the patient's home setting as needed to maintain their safety and comfort.

12. Attend educational lectures or seminars on providing care for cancer patients to learn more about the subject.

13. Talk about the patient's wishes for care at the end of life and confirm that their advance directives are in order.

To successfully manage side effects, adapt your approach to patient care to their particular requirements and side effects, and communicate often with the healthcare team.

The Cancer Support Community, Caregiver Action Network, Family Caregiver Alliance, National Alliance for Caregiving, Respite Care Services, Self-Care, Education, Task Delegation, Professional Support, Legal and Financial Planning, Government Assistance, Time Management, Staying Informed, Supportive Friends and Family, and Technology are among the resources and advice available to caregivers to help them maintain their well-being while providing care to someone with prostate cancer.

Prioritizing one's own health and requesting assistance when necessary are essential components of effective care for a loved one with prostate cancer. Communication with healthcare professionals is essential, and caregivers should be ready to share information, respect the patient's wishes, advocate on their behalf, keep things organized, use technology, think about hiring a medical advocate, and remain knowledgeable about the patient's condition and available treatments.

Caretakers need to be aware of the patient's health insurance coverage, check that providers are in network, keep records, and grasp the prerequisites for preauthorization and referrals in order to handle the financial and insurance elements of prostate cancer treatment. Additionally, they want to look into financial aid programs provided by hospitals, pharmaceutical firms, or nonprofit groups. Financial counselors may aid with insurance and give information on available financial resources, while prescription assistance programs can provide prescriptions at a reduced or free cost.

Medical expenditures may be paid for through budgeting for travel costs, investigating job benefits, and determining eligibility for government assistance programs like Medicaid or Social Security Disability Benefits. consulting a lawyer or financial adviser who specializes in healthcare-related issues for legal and financial guidance, particularly in cases of complicated financial circumstances. It's crucial to research charities that help men with prostate cancer since some charitable organizations provide financial assistance to cancer sufferers.

Carefully planning your budget is vital since it accounts for things like daily living expenditures, medical bills, and any changes in income brought on by caring. Patients should be urged to draft an advance directive or name a financial power of attorney to handle their finances in the event that they are unable to do it themselves. Advance preparedness is suggested. Keeping up with changes in healthcare legislation and insurance regulations that may affect coverage and pricing is also essential.

In conclusion, providing appropriate care for a loved one with prostate cancer necessitates putting one's own health first and enlisting the assistance of financial experts, patient advocates, or support groups. Caregivers may assure better treatment and results for their loved one with prostate cancer by using these suggestions.

II

"It's okay to feel overwhelmed sometimes. Caring for a loved one with prostate cancer is a lot to handle. Just take things one day at a time."

Impacts Of Caregiving to you

Giving care may be a difficult and emotionally taxing experience for people. It may result in tension, worry, guilt, melancholy, sorrow, and identity loss. Caretakers should identify their emotions, establish limits, get assistance, practice self-compassion, prioritize self-care, and make time for enjoyable and relaxing activities.

Self-care practices on a regular basis may support good physical and mental health. Physical health issues include fatigue, lack of sleep, self-care neglect, depression, and social isolation. Caretakers may disregard their own medical requirements, which might result in illnesses being unrecognized or untreated. Stress and anxiety, sadness, and social isolation are some of the mental health problems that people who are always concerned about the welfare of a loved one experience.

Regular checkups, adequate sleep, a healthy diet, regular exercise, delegation of tasks, realistic expectations, use of respite care services, connection with others, seeking professional mental health support, effective time management, and future planning are all methods for maintaining wellbeing.

1.Set your health as a top priority by scheduling routine checkups and attending to your personal requirements without disregarding any physical symptoms or indicators of stress.

2. receive enough sleep: Make sure you receive enough sleep by asking family members for assistance or by hiring a respite caregiver.

3. Eat a balanced diet and exercise often to maintain energy levels and lower stress.

4. Delegate and ask for assistance: Don't be afraid to ask for assistance from loved ones, friends, or trained carers.

5. Establish reasonable goals: Prioritize your duties based on significance and acknowledge that you can't complete everything flawlessly.

6. To give yourself frequent breaks and avoid burnout, use respite care services.

7. Remain socially connected by contacting friends and relatives for emotional support or signing up for caregiver support groups.

8. Seek professional mental health support:
Therapy or counseling may help you learn effective
coping mechanisms if you're battling with stress,
anxiety, or depression.

9. Time management: Plan your caregiving tasks
ahead of time and arrange time for yourself to take
breaks.

10. Make a long-term care plan for a loved one to
make sure their needs are addressed and lessen
future stress.

It is not selfish to take care of oneself; doing so is
necessary for both your health and your capacity to
care for your loved one effectively. Maintaining
your physical and emotional health requires
striking a balance between caring obligations and
self-care.

Setting boundaries is an essential part of caring
because it reduces burnout, protects health,
preserves identity, fosters emotional wellbeing,
strengthens bonds with others, and enhances the
quality of care. These limits improve the caregiver's
well-being as well as those of their loved one by
lowering stress, fostering better communication,

upholding dignity, assuring quality time, fostering independence, and fostering good connections.

Financial repercussions for caregivers might include decreased income, more spending, an effect on retirement, and even the possibility of debt. Caregivers should make a caring budget, look into financial assistance programs, speak with a financial adviser, think about long-term care insurance, and work with an attorney to draft the required legal papers in order to assure their financial security. Flexible work schedules, emergency savings, and tax breaks and deductions may all help caregivers preserve their income.

Open and honest talks about financial obligations and possible contributions to caregiving expenses need regular family financial discussions. Striking a balance between caring obligations and financial stability is crucial. Seeking expert advice and investigating the resources available can help you make educated choices, safeguard your financial wellbeing, and care for your loved one.

Caregivers may better care for their loved one and preserve their own well-being by establishing limits. They have the freedom to take breaks, refuel, and pursue their own hobbies, which may improve their relationships and general wellbeing.

Reduced income, higher costs, an impact on retirement savings, and a risk for debt are just a few of the financial effects of providing care. Caregivers should create a clear budget, look into financial assistance programs, speak with a financial adviser, think about long-term care insurance, and get legal and financial planning advice from an attorney to assure financial stability.

Effective financial management for carers may be facilitated by flexible employment arrangements, emergency savings, and tax benefits and deductions. Family financial conversations may ensure that members are aware of their financial obligations and may contribute to the expenses of providing care.

In order to preserve their own wellbeing and offer their loved ones the best care possible, carers must establish limits. Caregivers may make sure they are giving their loved ones the best care possible by setting up clear boundaries, requesting financial aid, and keeping a sound financial future.

Caregiving may have a substantial negative influence on social life and relationships, resulting in loneliness, relationship stress, independence loss, and less social chances. Caregivers should be open about their needs, plan respite time, join support groups, set reasonable expectations, assign tasks, use technology, organize social activities, seek professional assistance as needed, respect their own needs, and inform others about the caregiving role in order to maintain a support network.

It may be difficult to juggle work and caring obligations without experiencing professional setbacks, stagnant growth, financial hardship, and a skills gap. Caregiving balancing may cause income to decline, impacting retirement planning and financial security. Long absences from the workplace might also lead to stale expertise in the industry.

Open communication with their employer about flexible work arrangements, a clear separation of work and caregiving hours, the use of paid time off, an examination of employer benefits, preparation for emergencies, delegation of tasks, consideration of remote work, continuing professional development, consultation with a financial advisor, placing a high priority on self-care and stress management, and seeking support from caregiver support groups or professional counseling are all ways that caregivers can successfully balance work and caregiving.

Remote employment alternatives are worth looking into for caregivers as they provide greater freedom in juggling professions and caring. Even if they are on a lesser scale, they should look for chances to network and expand their skills. Planning ahead financially is important because it makes it easier to handle money, especially retirement funds, while providing care.

To prevent burnout and maintain a healthy lifestyle, self-care is crucial. A healthy person is better able to manage caregiving and employment commitments.

The burden of juggling work and caring is difficult, but it is manageable with careful preparation, honest communication, and a network of friends and family. Finding the ideal balance is crucial for one's job, as well as for their personal health and the quality of care they can provide to a loved one.

Burnout and guilt play a crucial part in caring since they may have a negative influence on the wellbeing of carers. Many things, including missed expectations, self-neglect, inadequacy, tough choices, persistent stress, a lack of support, and excessive demands, may lead to guilt.

Caregivers may exercise self-compassion by recognizing their limits and giving it their best effort in order to deal with guilt and exhaustion. They need to manage their time effectively, delegate tasks, ask for help, join support groups, seek professional assistance, communicate openly with loved ones about their limitations and feelings, utilize respite care services, set reasonable expectations, respect their needs, research legal and financial planning, and make future plans.

Routines of self-compassion and self-care are essential for carers because they lessen guilt and shame, boost resilience, improve mental health, deepen relationships, and avoid burnout. Treating oneself kindly and compassionately may help to relieve stress, anxiety, and sadness while also encouraging greater mental health. Additionally, it increases resiliency, assisting caregivers in overcoming difficulties and disappointments.

Self-care practices are crucial for reducing burnout, preserving physical and mental health, raising the standard of care, offering desperately needed pauses, and fostering independence. Practice mindfulness, set boundaries, get support, prioritize sleep, eat well, exercise frequently, stay connected, explore self-compassion exercises, use respite care services, and get professional help if you need it as self-compassion and self-care strategies.

By using mindfulness practices, caregivers may remain present and experience less stress. limits may be established and self-care activities can be given priority by setting clear limits and expressing requirements to others. Prioritizing sleep is crucial for preserving time and energy, and eating a balanced diet helps one stay physically well and have enough energy. Regular physical exercise helps lower stress and preserve physical health.

Maintaining social relationships may help with emotional support and battle feelings of loneliness. Caregiver exploration of self-compassion activities may be aided by self-compassion exercises such as sending compassionate letters or using positive affirmations. Using respite care services may provide frequent, guilt-free pauses for self-care.

In order to further explore self-compassion or self-care, it might be beneficial to seek therapy or counseling. Remember, exercising self-compassion and taking care of oneself is not selfish; it is necessary for caregivers' wellbeing and their capacity to provide their loved ones high-quality care. As a caregiver, you are making a worthwhile investment in their physical and emotional well.

As a caregiver, seeking professional assistance or therapy has several advantages for both the caregiver and the person they are caring for. These advantages include emotional support, stress reduction, conflict resolution, improved coping mechanisms, improved self-care, support for grieving and loss, education and resources, planning for respite, a reduction in caregiver burden, improved well-being, improved care quality, prevention of burnout, and a strengthening of bonds between caregivers and their loved ones.

Counseling is a useful way to deal with the different feelings that caregivers often experience, including stress, worry, despair, and guilt. Caregiver stress reduction and improved mental health may be achieved with the use of counseling strategies including stress management and relaxation exercises. Conflict resolution may aid family members in understanding one another, assist caregivers negotiate problems, and enhance communication.

Counseling also teaches better coping mechanisms, such as how to deal with challenging behaviors, make difficult choices, and handle difficulties associated with caring. Counselors may assist in prioritizing self-care and establishing boundaries so that caregivers can preserve their own wellbeing while providing care for a loved one. Support for grieving and loss is also offered for palliative or end-of-life care.

Counselors provide clients information and tools to aid in decision-making about a loved one's illness, available treatments, and support services. Planning for respite is another vital component of caring, as experts help carers organize their time off to relax and refuel.

In order to preserve caregivers' wellbeing while providing care for a loved one, respite care is very important. It gives them a much-needed break from their duties, lowering the likelihood of exhaustion and stress, promoting better care, fostering stronger relationships, offering a change of perspective, supporting independence, offering peace of mind, encouraging better decision-making, and improving the sustainability of long-term caregiving.

In-home care, adult day care programs, or brief stays in assisted living facilities are just a few examples of the many forms that respite care may take. To provide their loved one with the greatest care possible, carers must understand the importance of respite care and include it in their caring plans.

Finally, seeking professional assistance or therapy as a caretaker is not a show of weakness but rather a proactive move towards preserving their wellbeing and giving their loved one the best care possible. Caregivers may benefit from respite care and provide their loved ones with the finest care possible by including it in their caregiving plans.

How to Maintain Balance when being a caregiver

In order to preserve their physical health, mental stability, interpersonal connections, avoid burnout, provide an example of good behavior, improve decision-making, and guarantee long-term sustainability, carers of men with prostate cancer must engage in self-care activities. To discuss their thoughts and experiences, caregivers should turn to friends, relatives, or support groups.

Establish reasonable expectations and order work according to importance. Make time for self-care in your caregiving routine, even for little breaks. Reduce stress and increase your ability to remain calm in stressful circumstances by practicing relaxation methods like deep breathing, meditation, or yoga.

To feel more in control and to experience less worry, educate yourself regarding prostate cancer and the available treatments. To learn what to anticipate, talk to the medical staff. Delegate your chores to others, who may be eager to help with caring, and accept their assistance. Establish regular rest and recharge times; even a little stroll or some time alone may be reviving.

To provide short-term relief while seeing to your loved one's requirements, think about hiring respite care services. To minimize isolation and higher levels of stress, maintain social relationships outside of parenting. If stress becomes unbearable, seek professional assistance since counseling may teach useful coping mechanisms.

Openly discussing your emotions and limits with your loved one requires mindful conversation. They could have knowledge or be prepared to make changes to lessen stress. Always keep in mind that stress management is a continuous process and that what works for one person may not work for another. Try out several approaches to see which ones work best for you. Making self-care a priority is not selfish; it is necessary for keeping your health and giving your loved one with prostate cancer the best treatment possible.

Caregiver routines that include self-care activities are essential for men with prostate cancer. This entails getting up early, engaging in a self-care routine, eating a healthy breakfast, catering to your loved one's morning requirements, pausing for a while, and then eating a balanced lunch. You should continue to provide care and support throughout the afternoon, such as meal preparation or mobility aid, as necessary. Schedule respite care if it is offered.

Spend time with your loved one, have a nutritious dinner together, and do something enjoyable in the evening. As required, help your loved one take their medications and get ready for bed at night. After your loved one has relaxed, spend some time by yourself reading a book or having a nice bath.

Think back on your day, be thankful for the good times, and make plans for the caring duties for the next day before you go to bed. You must get a good night's sleep in order to be relaxed and ready to face the difficulties of the following day.

To fit your unique situation and your loved one's demands, modify this program. As caring often entails unanticipated events, flexibility is essential. To preserve your physical and mental wellbeing while giving your loved one with prostate cancer the best care possible, regularly evaluate your requirements for self-care and change as required.

The nature of their job often presents considerable emotional difficulties for caregivers of men with prostate cancer. These difficulties include anxiety and stress, loneliness and depression, guilt and burnout, loss and sorrow, annoyance and anger, doubt, role conflict, identity loss, and coping with end-of-life choices.

Caregivers may use stress-reduction tactics, enlist the aid of friends, family, or support networks, and maintain relationships with friends and family to preserve their mental health. If they have chronic depressive symptoms, they may also think about seeking counseling.

Due to the ongoing duties of caring, caregivers may feel guilty about taking time for themselves or develop burnout. Prioritizing the understanding that self-care is crucial for one's wellbeing and capacity to offer care. When it's feasible, assigning chores to others and getting respite care may both be beneficial. While irritation and fury may be handled via patience and understanding, sadness and rage can be experienced through grief therapy or support groups.

Caretakers should be aware of their loved one's health, concentrate on what they can manage, and acknowledge that certain things are beyond their control since uncertainty may be emotionally tiring. Setting limits and letting their employer know about their requirements can help carers avoid role tension and conflict that may arise from juggling caring with personal and professional obligations.

Finally, carers need to keep up their interests and pastimes that help them feel like themselves. Caretakers could be engaged in making tough end-of-life choices if prostate cancer advances to an advanced stage. It might be beneficial to have frank discussions with their loved one about their preferences and to seek advice from their medical staff.

For both the patient and the caregiver, getting help from others while providing care for men with prostate cancer is very important. It promotes emotional resilience, lessens social isolation, gives information and direction, offers respite and relief, facilitates decision-making, builds relationships, has an influence on one's own well-being, and enables greater life balance.

In conclusion, asking for help from friends, family, support groups, or medical experts is not a sign of weakness but rather a wise and considerate decision that helps the prostate cancer patient as well as the caregiver. Reaching out for assistance makes the shared path of caregiving more bearable and less taxing.

It might be difficult, but balancing caregiving duties with personal obligations and employment is crucial for overall wellbeing. Prioritize self-care, set reasonable expectations, manage time well, accept help from loved ones, friends, or support networks, communicate clearly, seek work-life balance, use technology and resources, routinely review your caregiving plan, practice self-compassion, uphold boundaries, and use respite care as necessary if you want to keep this balance.

1. Make self-care a priority by getting adequate sleep, eating well, and exercising often. Allocate time for fun pursuits and interests.

2. Establish reasonable goals for your caring, personal, and professional obligations, and develop the ability to refuse requests when required.

3. Using tools like calendars or apps, make a daily or weekly plan that allots time for caring duties, private pursuits, and work requirements.

4. Assign caring chores and obligations to family members, friends, or other support networks and accept their assistance.

5. To get understanding and support, communicate clearly with your employer, coworkers, and family members.

6. Ask your employer for flexible work schedule options, such as telecommuting or modifying working hours to fulfill caring obligations.

7. Make use of resources and technologies, including adult daycare facilities, support groups, and respite care services.

8. Reassess your caregiving schedule and strategy on a regular basis when your loved one's requirements change. To make the most of your caregiving strategy, think about getting expert advice from social workers or care coordinators.

9. Exercise self-compassion by being kind with yourself and learning to forgive yourself when you make errors or get frustrated.

10. Keep your caregiving function separate from your personal life or career, concentrating on one role as much as you can.

11. When required, use respite care services; it is an essential component of caring. To protect your wellbeing while giving your loved one the best care possible, keep in mind that finding a balance between caregiving, personal life, and job is a constant process.

Effective care requires maintaining physical health while tending to a patient with prostate cancer. Prioritizing preventive healthcare, staying hygienic, managing stress, preventing burnout, prioritizing preventive healthcare, maintaining medication and medical records, staying connected, seeking professional help, and comprehending the patient's needs and preferences are all ways to maintain physical health.

To make up for missed sleep, which is necessary for both physical and mental health, taking short naps throughout the day is a good idea. For optimal health, eat a well-balanced diet that is high in fruits, vegetables, lean meats, whole grains, and healthy fats. Additionally, regular exercise may enhance your mood and general wellbeing.

Practice stress-reduction methods like progressive muscle relaxation, deep breathing, or meditation to manage stress. Taking frequent breaks and planning time for oneself, whether it be through respite care services or asking friends and family for assistance, are important for preventing burnout. It's also critical to maintain appropriate personal hygiene routines, such as consistent handwashing, healthy eating, and vaccine updates.

Scheduling and attending routine health examinations and screenings, including cancer examinations if necessary, are part of preventive healthcare. It's critical to keep your healthcare provider up to date on your role as a caregiver. It's important to lift carefully, and using the right body mechanics and assistance equipment will help you avoid being hurt.

To preserve general health and avoid caregiver burnout, it is essential to keep track of medications and medical data. Involving others in caring may ensure everyone is on the same page and reduce burnout.

Problem-solving, ensuring safety, advocating for the patient, establishing boundaries between caregiving duties and personal life, minimizing misunderstandings, adapting to changing needs, maintaining emotional wellbeing, and peacefully resolving conflicts all depend on effective communication.

In conclusion, excellent communication is the key to providing successful treatment for men with prostate cancer. It helps the caregiver to provide the greatest care, preserve their own wellbeing, and create an atmosphere that is encouraging and empathetic. To preserve equilibrium and harmony in this demanding job, regular and open contact with healthcare professionals, the patient, and support networks is crucial.

Setting limits and asking for assistance are essential behaviors for carers to adopt because they safeguard their wellbeing, maintain interpersonal relationships, and enhance the quality of care delivered. They also ensure that caregivers set aside time and effort for self-care, which helps to avoid burnout.

By making sure that caregivers maintain their physical and emotional health, asking for assistance may help avoid burnout. Because several caregivers may share tasks and provide more thorough assistance, it often leads to better care for the patient.

Another advantage of asking for assistance is that it enables carers to take much-needed pauses, relax, and refuel. It may also help to share emotional support with friends or support groups to lessen stress and feelings of loneliness. Experts and professionals may provide advice on caregiving duties including dispensing drugs or providing specialized care.

Making caring decisions in collaboration with others might result in better informed judgments since they can get insight from their views and experiences. By fostering stronger bonds and a feeling of shared responsibility, family members and friends are better able to help the patient as a unit. Task delegation enables caregivers to concentrate on certain abilities or attention while giving ordinary work to others.

In conclusion, establishing clear limits and seeking assistance are effective ways that help both patients and caregivers. It may be very beneficial for both caregivers and patients to have a positive mindset while providing care for men with prostate cancer. A positive outlook can improve self-efficacy, foster better communication, foster better care, improve patient mood, increase resilience, decrease burnout risk, serve as a role model for the patient, foster a supportive environment, and help manage stress and anxiety.

In conclusion, keeping a positive viewpoint while providing care for a patient with prostate cancer may have a big influence on the experience, promoting mental health, improving the standard of care, and creating a welcoming and resilient caring environment. A optimistic outlook may significantly improve both the lives of caregivers and patients.

"Take care of yourself, too. Caring for someone else can be emotionally and physically draining. Make sure you're taking time for yourself to relax and recharge."
